Morton's Neuroma
My Success Story and What You Should Know

Shane Lemons

Copyright *Shane Michael Lemons 2018*

ALL RIGHTS RESERVED.

This book is protected by the copyright laws of the United States of America. This book may not be copied or reprinted for commercial gain or profit. There are no paid brand endorsements regarding products discussed. All opinions and advice are that of the author.

ISBN-13: 978-1724745972

ISBN-10: 1724745972

Table of Contents:

Chapter 1: Intro & Disclaimer..7

Chapter 2: My Story...11

Chapter 3: Conventional vs. Natural......................................19

Chapter 4: Successes...23

Chapter 5: What Did Not Work..27

Chapter 6: Footwear Basics...31

Chapter 7: Shoes to Consider..35

Chapter 8: In Closing - Four Years Later................................39

Chapter 1:
Intro & Disclaimer

This book and the entire contents are related to my own personal experience, and none of the information contained within is being shared as a personal prescription to you, and I am not responsible for any outcome you experience.

As always, you need to discuss all health issues and questions with your trusted physician(s), and then pursue what you feel is best for your situation.

It is my sincere hope that my story and the details coming up in this book will help you to think deeper about Morton's Neuroma, give you better insight into the anatomy of your foot, and give you a better view of options that exist beyond the generic answers you might have been given at this point. Also, Like, Share and stay up to date with even more info at facebook.com/beatingmn/! There is great content there, but I also try to update people with companies and products that should be avoided or researched further if they seem legit.

When I first realized I had MN, I became very frustrated with the enormous lack of info on how to *really* heal it without surgery. All I found was people complaining about how their surgery left them in worse pain, or how their orthotics didn't work, etc. No one had an answer for something really effective. So, me being me, I decided I wasn't going to settle for that. I had the hope that there had to be a really good *and* more natural way to go about this than just cutting back the nerve, taking pain killers, and using orthotics the rest of your life.

If you personally don't have a Morton's Neuroma, but you know someone who does, please share this information with him or her. As small as a Morton's Neuroma is, physically, it can be severe enough to where the person could be experiencing significantly decreased quality of life based on the lack of or ability to exercise, play, work, etc. I get messages from people all over the world, and many have no idea what to do. I truly believe this info will be of great value for those feeling hopeless with MN.

That's it for the intro. I hope you enjoy the book!

Chapter 2:
My Story

As I've found by my blog stats (which is not very up to date since I post just about everything to our Facebook page), many people across the globe suffer from Morton's Neuroma. When it hit me several years ago, I literally had no idea why the pain in my foot was not going away, nor had I ever even heard of a Morton's Neuroma to even think of that term as a possible cause. I also had no idea about how muddy the journey was going to be as I worked on finding my way out of the proverbial MN woods.

Before we get much further, this is a good spot for me to share a bit about myself for some history and better context:

- Past high school (football & track) and college athlete (football)
- Weight training and physically fit all my life from 5th grade to present
- Multiple broken bones, teeth, dislocations, you name it
- College weight of 255 lbs. (Lean enough to dunk a basketball)
- Post-college weight of a 205 - 215 lbs.
- Personal Trainer for several years
- Spent time in the Surgical field, with an above average knowledge of anatomy and physiology
- At the time of this book, I'm 41 years old

So, here's the timeline of my story that has already gained global attention on my blog and Facebook page @beatingmn:

While living in the Kansas City area, there was a gym near my office, so on my lunch break I would go work out for about 45 minutes about 3 days per week. The nice part with this gym was that it had an indoor track upstairs, and in Kansas City you do not want to be running outside in the winter. The track inside the gym, however, was bare concrete. Not ideal, but better than running outside in zero degrees, snow, or ice.

Shortly before joining this gym I had purchased a pair of major brand cross training shoes. Nothing fancy, really. They had a lot of cushion in the heal, so when I joined the gym I thought, "These will be perfect for running on that concrete track!" Big mistake, as I was soon to find out, but this is how most of us are programmed to think about shoe cushion (the more the better). More on that later.

Fast forward to a couple months into the gym membership and running in the shoes on that indoor track. At this time, the shoes had been getting a lot of pounding on that concrete track, and for some reason, I started to get this odd pain in my left forefoot, up near the left and middle area. I didn't think much of it at first, and I tried taking ibuprofen along with applying an occasional ice pack. After those healing efforts did not work, I went to a local drug store and bought a small pad that was supposed to go on the insole of your shoe. This little pad gave me a slight amount of relief, so I was hoping that after wearing it for a week or so that my foot would be healed and all would be forgotten with this nagging pain.

Unfortunately, the pain stayed very consistent. And I went from having an odd pain in my left foot to now being ticked off with the frequent pain in my left foot. You see, I've always been a pretty tough guy and my body typically heals quickly. And if I'm sick, which is rare, it usually passes more quickly for me than for other people. But not this time. About 30 - 40 days now of this odd, nagging pain had been present, and it just lingered, even after trying to do standard treatment. If you're reading this, you probably know what I mean.

So, the next thing I know I'm on my smart phone and on my computer during all non-working hours to do research on this pain in my foot. Through my research, it became very apparent that I had a Morton's Neuroma, which I was actually unfamiliar with, even though I had worked with podiatrists in the past. However, I didn't just take my research and give myself a guaranteed diagnosis; I scheduled an appointment with a local podiatrist in the city and had him look at it.

I'll share the deeper details of that office visit later, but to get to the point, he tested my foot and confirmed what I thought. It was indeed a Morton's Neuroma.

And that's where things got more interesting. The journey was really just beginning, because, as is the case with many injuries like this, you must discover the root cause first if you want to really correct the situation and be healed. If you just try to mask the pain and "make do" you really haven't solved anything, and you can actually make things far worse.

I will tell you now, so you don't have to wait in anticipation - I am healed. 100%. The methodology and info I'm about to roll out for you should provide valuable insight into my personal recovery, but also give you info to think about as you or someone you know looks for healing and restoration.

So, let's jump in.

Chapter 3:
Conventional vs. Natural

During my research, I found a certain video on YouTube (and specific podiatrist) to be very profound in what he shared. Essentially, it opened up my mind in terms of really grasping the fact that there are shoes and foot healing methods that are not getting the coverage they deserve, unlike the conventional and standard info where it's all about a global brand or procedure that can have a high billable rate with insurance. This is where a lightbulb moment occurred for me.

So often we end up just taking conventional medicine as absolute truth. We, as people, consumers, patients, etc. need to always ask, "Is this the best, or is this just the current norm, in terms of my overall health and long term victory over this health problem?" I encourage you to ask yourself and your doctor these things. There's nothing wrong with challenging the thoughts and norms of Western medicine and practices.

Anyway, the video I mentioned dives into the reality of how important it is to question the conventional approach, and look at the origins of foot problems, and what can be done to help reverse the problems.

I hope you take the time to watch it yourself (go to YouTube and watch the video titled "Origin of Natural Footcare with Dr. Ray McClanahan"). You can tell right away, based on how transparent and vulnerable this podiatrist is, that he really cares about natural and effective healing. Many doctors have a factory line mentality of speed and profit margin as their main goal, which has really damaged public health in my option. When it all becomes about the dollars and lifelong customers, it depletes the public trust, but it also creates massive problems for the patients/customers due to the quantities of drug prescriptions being handed out, all the while avoiding the root cause.

Chapter 4:
My Successes

As I touched on earlier, when I was trying to find legitimate info online as to what people were doing to actually reverse and/or heal Morton's Neuroma, I was coming up empty. It was extremely frustrating. Most of the searches yielded results of pay per click ads for podiatrists, surgery, and orthotics. And the non-ad results were typically a peppered mix of local podiatrists and health blogs with ticked off people that had either had surgery but ended up with what's called a "stump neuroma" or they simply haven't had surgery yet because they wanted to try steroid injections, orthotics, etc.

It was at this time that I decided to create a blog about my journey, and it's still up to this day, with monthly traffic from literally all over the world. On the blog, I had broken things down into what was working and what was not working, so everyone could see first-hand what I was doing.

So, I'll start with what worked for me:

- Getting rid of all of my conventional shoes (which I hated, but was worth it) that had elevated heels, constricting toe boxes, and too much toe spring
- Buying and wearing zero-drop flip flops or "toe shoes" for proper toe

splay

- Using quality toe spacers while I was at my office and at home (I was able to wear open sandals at work at this point)
- Lower leg stretching and rolling my feet over a golf ball while sitting
- Paying attention to my gait and foot strike position
- Using a metatarsal pad in the early stages of healing
- Sclerosing or otherwise known as dehydrated alcohol injections (in my early research, this seemed to have very high success rates among various populations, especially runners, and it was a huge factor, I believe, in my recovery. Unfortunately, many podiatrists do not offer this unless you ask them...it's almost as if they don't want you to know about it as an option)

For me, these items were synergistic in terms of their combined benefits. Keep in mind, this took quite a bit of time to come up with, but the beauty comes in the end. And hopefully these are things you can review, given your current stage of NM.

Chapter 5:
What Did Not Work

OK, so here is the reality, at least for me, of what did not work in dealing with or improving my Morton's Neuroma over the 5-6 months when I was in the early stage of the fight for recovery. The major thing I learned through all of this is that nerve injuries are far different than anything I have dealt with, whether broken bones, broken teeth, torn ligaments, strained muscles, or dislocated fingers.

It's my opinion that nerve issues need addressed immediately or else you are going to end up in a corner with what I see as only two ways out - surgery or alcohol injections. Now, this is MY list. It does not mean these practices won't work for you, but I tried each of these with no positive results to heal or restore the MN:

- Cold Laser Therapy - I spent a couple hundred dollars on this at a local Chiropractor's Office (awesome Chiro office and team, just no benefit from this specific treatment plan).
- Crutches - Yes, I put myself on crutches to see if it would help reduce the MN. I did a total of about 14 days. Literally no improvement there.
- Anti-inflammatory / Ibuprofen - Nada. It's my theory and experience that if the NM is too enlarged and thickened up that this method won't do anything but jack up your liver and stomach.

- Icing - So, here's the thing with MN; the position is above the fat pad on the foot, so it is very difficult to get the ice to really hit the right spot. You can try from the dorsal position, but again, if the MN is too advanced, it seems like wasted time and energy, and it didn't help at all.
- Elevation - Same deal. If your MN has several weeks behind it, it might be too late.
- Orthotics - I'll admit that I did not try any custom orthotics in terms of purchasing any, because, to me, that is just masking the problem anyway, and it's counterintuitive to your foot's design to spread when you walk. And frankly, I don't want to spend $500 on this "remedy" in which I am just putting my feet back into the problem causing item (constriction). Just putting an orthotic into narrow shoes again does nothing for real restoration of the nerve or the root cause. I did try one on in an orthotic shop, and immediately I could tell it was not the answer due to immediate pain it gave me.

So, that's my experience with those avenues. I'm glad I tried them, but hopefully I can save you the time, money, and energy that those methods consume!

Chapter 6:
Footwear Basics

So, if we are going to be serious about addressing Morton's, or any other foot or toe condition for that matter, we need to seriously look at a few pieces related to the cause. As much of the research showed when I really dug in, many of the cultures around the globe that have little to no foot problems are those that are barefoot or wear minimal footwear, such as thin, wide sandals. And it makes sense - if you look at a baby's feet, the feet are usually wide, and the parents are usually only seeing and buying shoes in the stores that are wide in the toe box. And those shoes are usually close to zero drop.

Unfortunately, in our society here in America and many other "developed" countries, fashion has been winning out over health. As we get out of our toddler years, we start putting our feet into shoes that look cool, feel comfortable at first, and even seem like they have "science" on their side due to advertising. However, if you ask any podiatrist that has been keeping up with shoe and foot issues in America or any other modernized culture, they will tell you (if they are honest) what is really going on and how many shoes today are <u>not</u> made with forefoot expansion models of 15%+ or with toe boxes that are not stressing the inter-digital nerve areas by pre-formed toe spring. If you've seen the movie "A Perfect Storm" you get some idea of what we're doing to our feet via our conventional shoes. So, with that, here's a more thorough list of what to consider:

- The size of your foot AND toes while relaxed and standing and even running, vs the size of the shoe that you are trying to make it fit into
- The toe spring (try to avoid shoe molds where your toes aim upward)
- The heel height vs the toe box level (try to keep at a "zero-drop")
- The landing or strike created when you walk or run in the shoe
- The amount of room in the toe box (make sure it's roomy)

Here's one way to test that I read about online that seems to make a ton of sense. If you are in the market for shoes, just take the insole out of the shoe, place the insole on the ground, and then step on top of the insole (barefoot is best). If the toe box is too narrow, you will know immediately because your toes will be falling over the sides of the insole when you have all of your weight on it. You'll know you have enough room in the toe box when the shoe's insole is wider than your forefoot when you're stepping on it. In other words, you'll see the edges of the insole, still, even when you're stepping on it with all of your weight.

Chapter 7:
Shoes to Consider

During all of my research on shoes that are more naturally fitting to what the adult foot should be in, whether walking, running, hiking, etc., here is the list I have come across so far. Some of them I personally wear now, or have worn, and I can attest to the fit being wider than normal for a natural foot shape, zero drop, and little to no toe spring:

- Vivobarefoot (numerous models)

- Merrell (I stick with the Glove models only)
- Lems
- Vibram FiveFingers
- Note - there are several other legit brands out now, and others that are starting to pop up through crowdfunding campaigns, so I'll be reviewing these on our Facebook page as time permits

As for shopping, you're probably not going to find any of the products I have listed in the book at a local retailer. You might be able to find a couple shoe models at REI, but most of the time, I make my purchases on Amazon and eBay. You can also purchase directly from the company websites in most cases.

Now that you'll be shopping with a sharper eye, beware of the shoes that have too much cushion, heel height, narrow toe boxes and too much toe spring. Use the test described in the previous chapter as a guide. When looking at shoes, consider the following:

- Did it pass the insole test?
- Is the footbed too squishy at rest?
- When I walk in this shoe, are my toes allowed to naturally spread?
- Is the shoe zero drop?
- When I walk in this shoe, does it make my feet land in an unnatural position?

The answers to these questions will help determine if you should or should not invest in the product. And keep in mind, you want your toes to be free to splay while at rest and during activity, avoiding too much compression of the bones against the footwear or bone against bone. So, even if a pair of shoes look a bit crazy, still keep the main focus on foot health, not public approval on fashion. I've gotten plenty of stares with certain shoes I wear now, but given what I know, it doesn't phase me!

Chapter 8:
Four Years Later

As I finish writing this book, it has now been over 4 years since I restored my foot with my own combination/method, and my neuroma is not only gone, but there's literally no sign of it. I have zero pain. I have zero concern of it repeating. The reason? It's simple - I had the sclerosing done and I had gotten to the root issues with proper footwear and therefore the proper foot mechanics can function as they were designed. I'm not jamming my size 13 (US) foot into a poorly designed shoe, no matter what the brand name is or what popular person might endorse it. I'm aware of the brands that "get it" and I stick with them.

Not only is my foot restored, but so is my quality of life. I can run on any terrain I want to, I can play with my three lively boys without hesitation, I can do any type of weight training I want to, etc. And this is my hope and prayer for you. Your body was designed to be active, as you certainly know.

Hopefully, if you're reading this, you've gained information that you can review and consider in your journey. However, this material should not just be used if you currently have a Morton's Neuroma, but also as preventive care; it's valuable for everyone to know about, because everyone you know buys and wears shoes. I know I wish I had been told about natural foot care and proper footwear when I was younger.

It would have saved me a lot of time, money, guessing, and physical pain.

So, in closing, here is a recap of what you can do, literally right now, to get things aligned for foot health:

1.) Grab all of your shoes, and do the insole test
2.) If they don't "pass" then you need to get some that do so your foot can be in a zero drop and wide toe box environment
3.) Look into brands that can pass the questions in the previous chapter, shop around either online or a local retailer
4.) If necessary, use quality metatarsal pads in the meantime for pain relief (I preferred the foam ones with adhesive backing, so you can place them on your barefoot before putting a sock on)

5.) Look into purchasing quality toe spacers to get the toes back into better spacing distance from each other (I used a product called Correct Toes)

6.) If necessary, find a podiatrist that is more inline with natural foot healing

7.) Know your options - if you're being pressured to have a resection or other surgery, take the time to weigh every option (there's no way to reverse a resection surgery if the resection goes bad/wrong)

And here's the recap of my personal process:
- Research and self-diagnosed
- Confirmed diagnosis by podiatrist
- Focused on addressing the root cause
- Got rid of all poorly designed footwear
- Did 3 sclerosing injections at 1.5 week intervals

- In this time span, I was constantly wearing my toe spacers and the adhesive metatarsal pads in proper footwear and mostly open-toed sandals
- Avoided any excessive pounding or flexion in my forefoot for several months
- Kept a positive attitude

Also, here are some tips/pointers/suggestions:

- Always, always, ALWAYS get an actual diagnosis, not just an educated guess by a podiatrist. You must get confirmation that you're dealing with MN and not something else; the structure of the foot is beautifully complex, and as such, a myriad of injuries are possible. No guessing by you or your doctor.
- I've personally never come across a person with MN that had success with cortisone injections. My personal deduction is that

nerve tissue does not respond to steroids the same way muscular tissue does, and therefore it's not an adequate option.
- MN is very specific in location, so if you're having pain all over your foot, including your ankle or other places far from the metatarsals, you're likely dealing with something other than MN.
- Do not go through the sclerosing process unless you do the synergistic process I've noted above; if you get the sclerosing done but keep jamming your feet into crappy shoes, expect a crappy result. You must create the synergistic environment for healing (sclerosing, toe spacers, metatarsal pads, zero drop + wide toe box footwear only, and no pounding/running for a while). When you do these things together, you should start to see a difference after a few weeks.
- With the sclerosing injections, I was able to get 3 and that worked for me because I did other positive things mentioned above for a healthy healing environment. That said, I've heard of some people having up to 6 injections. I am pretty sure none of them

were doing the exact process I've come up with, and therefore took in more injections. That's my guess, anyway.

That's it, friends! Your foot health and MN might be easier to manage than you thought, and hopefully you can get things back where they belong.

Here's to a healthy future!